Copyright © 2020 by Verona Jackson

RND

All rights reserved. No part of this publication may be reproduced, distributed, or transmitted in any form or by any means, including photocopying, recording, or other electronic or mechanical methods, without the prior written permission of the publisher, except in the case of brief quotations embodied in critical reviews and certain other noncommercial uses permitted by copyright law

Table of Contents

Introduction 5

What Is Fatty Liver 6

   Alcoholic Fatty Liver Disease 8

   Nonalcoholic Fatty Liver Disease............ 9

      Diagnosis... 9

      Blood Tests... 10

      Imaging Procedures 11

Symptoms Of Fatty Liver 12

Causes of Fatty Liver Disease 14

What Should One Eat To Cure Fatty Liver Disease 15

6 Foods To Avoid If You Have A Fatty Liver 21

Clinical Trials 23

Lifestyle And Home Remedies 23

With your doctor's help, you can take steps to control your nonalcoholic fatty liver disease. You can: 23

Alternative Medicine 26

Preparing For Your Appointment 29

What You Can Do: 30

What To Expect From Your Doctor 33

Who Is At Risk For Fatty Liver Disease? 35

How Is Fatty Liver Disease Diagnosed 38

Fatty Liver Recipes 45

Mexican Fruit Salad 45

Pecan Granola Bars............................ 49

Quick, Budget-Friendly Homemade Oat Milk Recipe.. 54

No Bake Blueberry Energy Bites.......... 56

Fresh Corn Salsa (Chipotle Copycat).... 58

Baked Zucchini Fries............................ 60

Easy & Healthy Avocado Chicken Salad 62

Ginger Lemonade................................. 64

Delicious Chili-Lime Grilled Corn 67

Tuscan Vegetable Soup 69

Homemade Water Kefir Soda 72

The Ultimate Healthy Gingersnaps....... 76

Introduction

Liver is one of the most important organs of the body. Most of us know that it is responsible for filtering the blood coming from the digestive tract, before passing it to the rest of the body. It helps detoxify chemicals and metabolises drugs; while doing so, it secretes bile juice. Liver helps make proteins and is known to be important for blood clotting and other functions. It constantly helps in fighting various infections, removes toxins, controls cholesterol and regulates blood sugar. The body tends to store fat in various parts in the system that is used up as energy and insulation. The large meaty organ liver is partially made up of fat; however, if the fat content in this organ becomes too high, then the person may suffer from fatty liver.

What Is Fatty Liver

A fatty liver is caused when the carbohydrates or fats or both being regularly consumed is far more than what your liver can process. The excess fat is usually stored in your cells. Beyond a point, it begins to get stored in and around the liver resulting in a fatty liver condition." Fatty liver is when fat in the organ accounts for more than five to 10 percent of your liver's weight. It is a reversible condition that can be resolved with lifestyle modifications. It doesn't have peculiar symptoms that one can differentiate into this condition. However, if not diagnosed early, this condition may cause serious damage to the liver.

Fatty liver is of two types: alcoholic fatty liver disease and non-alcoholic fatty liver disease. It tends to damage the liver, inhibiting it from removing toxins and producing bile for the digestive system, two of which are the most important functions of the liver. If the most basic function of filtering out toxins is interrupted, there are chances of developing numerous health conditions.

Alcoholic Fatty Liver Disease

Alcoholic fatty liver disease, also called alcoholic steatohepatitis

One of the possible complications of this condition is steatohepatitis, which is the inflammation of the liver. This may lead to liver damage. A damaged liver may become hardened and scarred, which is a condition called cirrhosis. Cirrhosis can be a serious medical condition that may result in liver failure.

Nonalcoholic Fatty Liver Disease

Diagnosis

Because NAFLD causes no symptoms in most cases, it frequently comes to medical attention when tests done for other reasons point to a liver problem. This can happen if your liver looks unusual on ultrasound or if you have an abnormal liver enzyme test.

Tests done to pinpoint the diagnosis and determine disease severity include:

Blood Tests

- Complete blood count

- Liver enzyme and liver function tests

- Tests for chronic viral hepatitis (hepatitis A, hepatitis C and others)

- Celiac disease screening test

- Fasting blood sugar

- Hemoglobin A1C, which shows how stable your blood sugar is

- Lipid profile, which measures blood fats, such as cholesterol and triglycerides

Imaging Procedures

Imaging procedures used to diagnose NAFLD include:

- Abdominal ultrasound, which is often the initial test when liver disease is suspected.

- Computerized tomography (CT) scanning or magnetic resonance imaging (MRI) of the abdomen. These techniques lack the ability to distinguish NASH from NAFLD, but still may be used.

- Transient elastography, an enhanced form of ultrasound that measures the stiffness of your liver. Liver stiffness indicates fibrosis or scarring.

• Magnetic resonance elastography, works by combining MRI imaging with sound waves to create a visual map (elastogram) showing the stiffness of body tissues.

Symptoms Of Fatty Liver

As mentioned above, fatty liver has no particular associated symptoms. Some of the common symptoms may include fatigue or abdominal discomfort. Diagnosis may show an enlarged liver. Excess fat in the liver can cause inflammation, which can further cause symptoms including:

- Fatigue

- Confusion

- Abdominal pain

- Weight loss

- Loss of appetite

- Physical weakness

In severe cases, there are chances of developing an enlarged abdomen, jaundice and a tendency to bleed more easily.

Causes of Fatty Liver Disease

Nutritionist Ritesh Bawri says, "The most important cause of this disease seems to be obesity or diabetes as over 65% of people with diabetes also look to be reporting fatty liver." Another common cause of fatty liver disease is alcoholism or binge-drinking. Here are some other reasons that may cause the condition.

1. Obesity

2. Diabetes

3. Eating a high-fat and high-sugar diet

4. Genetic inheritance

5. Rapid weight loss

6. Side effects of medication

7. High levels of fat in the blood

What Should One Eat To Cure Fatty Liver Disease

Dietary habits are significantly associated with health state. A correct diet, associated with a healthy lifestyle may in fact contribute to the maintenance of a healthy human body. Similarly, the right dietary intake may help cure both alcoholic and non-alcoholic fatty liver diseases. According to Ritesh Bawri, "The best way to manage a fatty liver condition is to reduce processed foods, especially those high in sugar. Similarly, cutting back on flour and white sugar can help. Obviously, reducing or eliminating the intake of alcohol, which is nothing but sugar also helps. Eating plenty of good quality fruits and vegetables provides adequate nutrition to your body and also help you reduce the amount of fat. Finally, managing your calorie intake ensures that your energy requirement is in balance and the excess food is not stored as fat in and around your body."

According to a study published in the Medscape, the Mediterranean diet and a low-fat diet could help cure fatty liver disease along with physical exercises. Mediterranean diet includes the consumption of fresh fruits and vegetables, olive oil and fish and almost no meat. Mediterranean diet has been deemed as one of the healthiest diets that help keep various ailments at bay.

We suggest some foods that may help reverse the effects of fatty liver- They are:

1. Garlic

This kitchen ingredient may help cure fatty liver disease. According to a study published in Advanced Biomedical Research, garlic appears to help reduce body weight and fat in people with fatty liver disease.

2. Coffee

According to a report published in the Annals of Hepatology, coffee contains certain compounds that may help protect the body from non-alcoholic fatty liver disease. Adding coffee to the morning routine may be a great addition to a person's fatty liver diet.

3. Broccoli

According to a study published in the journal of Nutrition, long term consumption of broccoli helped prevent fat build-up in the liver of mice.

Cruciferous vegetables like spinach, cabbage, cauliflower are known to have a great impact on the liver.

4. Green Tea

Tea, according to World Journal of Gastroenterology, especially green tea has high levels of antioxidants that help reduce body fat percentage and fat in the blood.

5. Soy Or Whey Protein

Tofu may actually reduce fat build-up in the liver. Not just this, tofu has super-low fat content and high-protein that makes it even healthier for a fatty liver diet.

6. Walnuts

Foods rich in omega-3 fatty acids are great for liver health. A study found that eating walnuts improved liver function tests in people with non-alcoholic fatty liver disease.

7. Sunflower Seeds

These crunchy delights are excellent sources of vitamin E, an antioxidant, which helps protect the liver from further damage. So, include them in your fatty liver diet.

8. Olive Oil

The presence of omega-3 fatty acids in olive oil help lower liver enzymes levels and control weight. So, include this healthy oil in your fatty liver diet.

6 Foods To Avoid If You Have A Fatty Liver

There are definitely foods you should avoid or limit if you have fatty liver disease. These foods generally contribute to weight gain and increasing blood sugar.

The foods are as follows:

- **Alcohol.** Alcohol is a major cause of fatty liver disease as well as other liver diseases.

- **Added Sugar.** Stay away from sugary foods such as candy, cookies, sodas, and fruit juices. High blood sugar increases the amount of fat buildup in the liver.

- **Fried Foods.** These are high in fat and calories.

- **Salt.** Eating too much salt can make your body hold on to excess water. Limit sodium to less than 1,500 milligrams per day.

- **White Bread, Rice, And Pasta.** White usually means the flour is highly processed, which can raise your blood sugar more than whole grains due to a lack of fiber.

- **Red Meat.** Beef and deli meats are high in saturated fat

Clinical Trials

Explore Mayo Clinic studies testing new treatments, interventions and tests as a means to prevent, detect, treat or manage this disease.

Lifestyle And Home Remedies

With your doctor's help, you can take steps to control your nonalcoholic fatty liver disease. You can:

- **Lose Weight.** If you're overweight or obese, reduce the number of calories you eat each day and increase your physical activity in order to lose weight. Calorie reduction is the key to losing weight and managing this disease. If you have tried to lose weight in the past and have been unsuccessful, ask your doctor for help.

- **Choose A Healthy Diet.** Eat a healthy diet that's rich in fruits, vegetables and whole grains, and keep track of all calories you take in.

- **Exercise And Be More Active.** Aim for at least 30 minutes of exercise most days of the week. If you're trying to lose weight, you might find that more exercise is helpful. But if you don't already exercise regularly, get your doctor's OK first and start slowly.

- **Control Your Diabetes.** Follow your doctor's instructions to stay in control of your diabetes. Take your medications as directed and closely monitor your blood sugar.

- **Lower Your Cholesterol.** A healthy plant-based diet, exercise and medications can help keep your cholesterol and your triglycerides at healthy levels.

- **Protect Your Liver.** Avoid things that will put extra stress on your liver. For instance, don't drink alcohol. Follow the instructions on all medications and over-the-counter drugs. Check with your doctor before using any herbal remedies, as not all herbal products are safe.

Alternative Medicine

No alternative medicine treatments are proved to cure nonalcoholic fatty liver disease. But researchers are studying whether some natural compounds could be helpful, such as:

- **Vitamin E.** In theory, vitamin E and other vitamins called antioxidants could help protect the liver by reducing or neutralizing the damage caused by inflammation. But more research is needed.

Some evidence suggests vitamin E supplements may be helpful for people with liver damage caused by nonalcoholic fatty liver disease. But vitamin E has been linked with increased risk of death and, in men, an increased risk of prostate cancer.

- **Coffee.** In studies of people with nonalcoholic fatty liver disease, those who reported drinking two or more cups of coffee a day had less liver damage than those who drank little or no coffee. It's not yet clear how coffee may influence liver damage, but findings suggest it may contain certain compounds that may play a role in fighting inflammation.

If you already drink coffee, these results may make you feel better about your morning cup of coffee. But if you don't already drink coffee, this probably isn't a good reason to start. Discuss the potential benefits of coffee with your doctor.

Preparing For Your Appointment

Start by making an appointment with your family doctor or primary doctor if you have signs and symptoms that worry you. If your doctor suspects you may have a liver problem, such as nonalcoholic fatty liver disease, you may be referred to a doctor who specializes in the liver (hepatologist).

Because appointments can be brief, it's a good idea to be well prepared. Here's some information to help you get ready, and what to expect from your doctor.

What You Can Do:

- Be aware of any pre-appointment restrictions. When you make the appointment, be sure to ask if there's anything you need to do in advance, such as restrict your diet.

- Write down any symptoms you're experiencing, including any that may seem unrelated to the reason for which you scheduled the appointment.

- Make a list of all medications, vitamins or supplements that you're taking.

- Take any relevant medical records, such as records of any tests you've had that relate to your current condition.

- Take a family member or friend along. Sometimes it can be difficult to absorb all the information provided during an appointment. Someone who accompanies you may remember something that you missed or forgot.

- Write down questions to ask your doctor.

If you find out you have nonalcoholic fatty liver disease, some basic questions to ask include:

- Is the fat in my liver hurting my health?

- Will my fatty liver disease progress to a more serious form?

- What are my treatment options?

- What can I do to keep my liver healthy?

- I have other health conditions. How can I best manage them together?

- Should I see a specialist? Will my insurance cover it?

- Are there any brochures or other printed material that I can take with me? What websites do you recommend?

- Should I plan for a follow-up visit?

In addition to the questions that you've prepared to ask your doctor, don't hesitate to ask questions during your appointment.

What To Expect From Your Doctor

Your doctor is likely to ask you a number of questions, such as:

- Have you experienced any symptoms, such as yellowing of the eyes or skin and pain or swelling in your abdomen?

- If you had tests done at that time, what were the results?

- Do you drink alcohol?

- What medications do you take, including over-the-counter drugs and supplements?

- Have you ever been told that you have hepatitis?

- Do other people in your family have liver disease?

Who Is At Risk For Fatty Liver Disease?

The cause of nonalcoholic fatty liver disease (NAFLD) is unknown. Researchers do know that it is more common in people who

- Have type 2 diabetes and prediabetes

- Have obesity

- Are middle aged or older (although children can also get it)

- Are Hispanic, followed by non-Hispanic whites. It is less common in African Americans.

- Have high levels of fats in the blood, such as cholesterol and triglycerides

- Have high blood pressure

- Take certain drugs, such as corticosteroids and some cancer drugs

- Have certain metabolic disorders, including metabolic syndrome

- Have rapid weight loss

- Have certain infections, such as hepatitis C

- Have been exposed to some toxins

NAFLD affects about 25 percent of people in the world. As the rates of obesity, type 2 diabetes, and high cholesterol are rising in the United States, so is the rate of NAFLD. NAFLD is the most common chronic liver disorder in the United States.

Alcoholic fatty liver disease only happens in people who are heavy drinkers, especially those who have been drinking for a long period of time. The risk is higher for heavy drinkers who are women, have obesity, or have certain genetic mutations.

How Is Fatty Liver Disease Diagnosed

Because there are often no symptoms, it is not easy to find fatty liver disease. Your doctor may suspect that you have it if you get abnormal results on liver tests that you had for other reasons. To make a diagnosis, your doctor will use

- Your medical history

- A physical exam

- Various tests, including blood and imaging tests, and sometimes a biopsy

As part of the medical history, your doctor will ask about your alcohol use, to find out whether fat in your liver is a sign of alcoholic fatty liver disease or nonalcoholic fatty liver (NAFLD). He or she will also ask which medicines you take, to try to determine whether a medicine is causing your NAFLD.

During the physical exam, your doctor will examine your body and check your weight and height. Your doctor will look for signs of fatty liver disease, such as:

- An enlarged liver

- Signs of cirrhosis, such as jaundice, a condition that causes your skin and whites of your eyes to turn yellow

You will likely have blood tests, including liver function tests and blood count tests. In some cases you may also have imaging tests, like those that check for fat in the liver and the stiffness of your liver. Liver stiffness can mean fibrosis, which is scarring of the liver. In some cases you may also need a liver biopsy to confirm the diagnosis, and to check how bad the liver damage is.

What are the treatments for fatty liver disease?

Doctors recommend weight loss for nonalcoholic fatty liver. Weight loss can reduce fat in the liver, inflammation, and fibrosis. If your doctor thinks that a certain medicine is the cause of your NAFLD, you should stop taking that medicine. But check with your doctor before stopping the medicine. You may need to get off the medicine gradually, and you might need to switch to another medicine instead.

There are no medicines that have been approved to treat NAFLD. Studies are investigating whether a certain diabetes medicine or Vitamin E can help, but more studies are needed.

The most important part of treating alcohol-related fatty liver disease is to stop drinking alcohol. If you need help doing that, you may want to see a therapist or participate in an alcohol recovery program. There are also medicines that can help, either by reducing your cravings or making you feel sick if you drink alcohol.

Both alcoholic fatty liver disease and one type of nonalcoholic fatty liver disease (nonalcoholic steatohepatitis) can lead to cirrhosis. Doctors can treat the health problems caused by cirrhosis with medicines, operations, and other medical procedures. If the cirrhosis leads to liver failure, you may need a liver transplant.

What are some lifestyle changes that can help with fatty liver disease?

If you have any of the types of fatty liver disease, there are some lifestyle changes that can help:

- Eat a healthy diet, limiting salt and sugar, plus eating lots of fruits, vegetables, and whole grains

- Get vaccinations for hepatitis A and B, the flu and pneumococcal disease. If you get hepatitis A or B along with fatty liver, it is more likely to lead to liver failure. People with chronic liver disease are more likely to get infections, so the other two vaccinations are also important.

• Get regular exercise, which can help you lose weight and reduce fat in the liver

• Talk with your doctor before using dietary supplements, such as vitamins, or any complementary or alternative medicines or medical practices. Some herbal remedies can damage your liver.

Fatty Liver Recipes

Mexican Fruit Salad

Ingredients

- 1 1/4 cup dried unsulphured figs or about 5-6 ounces (stems cut off)
- 2 cups raw cashews
- 1 cup unsweetened coconut flakes (plus extra for topping)
- 1 tsp alcohol-free vanilla
- 1/4 tsp sea salt
- 1/3 to 2/3 cup or more of dark chocolate chips, to melt
- optional add-ins 1 tbsp protein powder, chia, nuts, cocoa powder.

Directions

1. Line a square baking pan with parchment paper. Set aside.
2. Next make sure your dried figs have all the stems cut off.
3. Place cashew, coconut, salt, vanilla, and figs in food processor. (If you don't have a high powered food processor or blender, then divide the ingredients in half and blend/grind in two batches).
4. Blend until mixture is fine and able to stick together well. See pictures above.
5. Pour mixture into baking dish and press down well.

6. While the fig/cashew mix sets in pan, melt your dark chocolate.

7. Place dark chocolate in a microwave safe bowl or on stove top. Heat until melted. About 60-90 seconds in microwave mixing half way. See notes for stove top option.

8. You can also use my homemade magic chocolate shell recipe if you want a thicker chocolate coat.

9. Next pour the chocolate over the cashew coconut batter and spread it evenly in the dish to cover all. noted if you need more dark chocolate to cover, just melt an additional 1/4 cup.

10. Optional topping – Sprinkle extra coconut, cashew, sliced fig, and dash of sea salt on top of chocolate (evenly).
11. Place in freezer for 20 minutes or fridge for a few hrs.
12. Once they are hardened, remove from fridge.
13. Slice into bars and wrap each one in foil for a quick grab and go bar. Or store in an airtight container.
14. Best kept in fridge for freshness. Feel free to freezer for up to 8-10 weeks. These really do keep well!

Pecan Granola Bars

Ingredients

- 1 1/4 cups pecan halves
- 2 cups quick-cooking oats
- 1 tsp ground cinnamon
- 1/2 tsp fine sea salt
- 1 cup homemade pecan butter or creamy almond butter or peanut butter
- 1/2 cup maple syrup or honey
- 1 1/2 tsp vanilla extract

Directions

1. Line a 9-inch square baker with one strip of parchment paper, cut to fit neatly across the

base. The parchment paper will make it easy for you to slice the bars later.

2. For maximum flavor, toast the pecans: In a medium skillet over medium heat, toast the pecans, stirring frequently (don't let them burn!), until they are nice and fragrant, about 4 to 7 minutes. Transfer them to a cutting board to cool. Set aside 16 of your prettiest pecan halves for garnish, then chop the rest. Set aside.

3. In a large mixing bowl, combine the oats, cinnamon, and salt, and stir to blend. Set aside.

4. If you have made pecan butter for this recipe*, add the maple syrup and vanilla to

your food processor or blender and blend to combine. If not, in a 2-cup liquid measuring cup, measure out 1 cup nut butter. Top with ½ cup maple syrup, followed by the vanilla extract. Whisk until well blended. (If you must, you can gently warm the liquid mixture in the microwave or on the stovetop.)

5. Pour the liquid ingredients into the dry ingredients. Use a big spoon to mix them together until the two are evenly combined and no dry oats remain. Add the chopped pecans and stir until they are evenly dispersed. The drier the mixture, the more firm the bars will be, so stir in extra oats if

the mixture seems wet. Conversely, if you used a super thick nut butter, you might need to drizzle in another tablespoon of honey to help it all stick together.

6. Transfer the mixture to the prepared square baker. Use your spoon to arrange the mixture fairly evenly in the baker. Cover the bottom of a flat, round surface (like a short, sturdy drinking glass) with a strip of parchment paper (see photo) and pack the mixture down as firmly and evenly as possible. Press the reserved pecan halves into the surface to create 4 even rows and 4 even columns (see photo).

7. Cover the baker and refrigerate for at least one hour, or overnight. This gives the oats time to absorb moisture so the granola bars can set. When you're ready to slice, lift the bars out of the baker by grabbing both both ends of the parchment paper. Use a sharp chef's knife to slice the mixture into 4 even rows and 4 even columns (these "bars" stick together better in a square shape).

8. For portability, you can wrap individual bars in plastic wrap or parchment paper. Bars keep well for a couple of days at room temperature, but I recommend storing individually wrapped bars in a freezer-safe

bag in the freezer for best flavor. They'll keep for several months in the freezer.

Quick, Budget-Friendly Homemade Oat Milk Recipe

Ingredients

- 1 cup gluten-free rolled oats*
- 4 cups water (use less water for thicker, creamier milk!)
- 1 pinch salt
- 1-2 whole dates, pitted or 1 tbsp maple syrup (optional, for making sweetened milk)
- 1/2 tsp pure vanilla extract (optional, for making sweetened vanilla oat milk)

Directions

1. Add oats, water, salt, and any additional ingredients to a high speed blender and blend until the mixture is well combined, about 45-seconds. (Avoid over-blending as it can make the milk slimy in texture.)
2. Pour the mixture through a sieve or over a large mixing bowl covered with cheesecloth or a very thin, clean kitchen towel to strain the oats from the milk. Remove the oat pulp from whatever you are using to strain the mixture and strain the milk a second time.
3. Pour your milk into a sealed container and refrigerate up to 5 days. Before using, shake well. Aside from using it in coffee,

tea, cereal, granola or smoothies, it can also be used in baked goods as well where milk is an ingredient. Avoid heating the milk separately though as it will cause the milk to become thick and gelatinous.

*While oats are gluten-free they can be processed on the same machines as gluten-containing grains contaminating the oats with enough gluten to cause a reaction in those with celiac.

No Bake Blueberry Energy Bites

Ingredients

- 2 cup raw old-fashioned oats
- 1/2 cup almond butter

- 1/2 cup honey
- 1 teaspoon alcohol-free vanilla
- 1/2 teaspoon cinnamon
- 1 cup dried blueberries

Directions

1. In a large bowl, mix together oats, almond butter, honey, vanilla, and cinnamon.
2. Next fold in the blueberries until they are evenly distributed in the mix.
3. Refrigerate mixture for 30-60 minutes, or until it becomes solidified.
4. Mold mixture into bite-sized balls and serve. You can keep the energy bites in an air tight

container in the refrigerator up to one week or freeze and defrost when needed.

Fresh Corn Salsa (Chipotle Copycat)

Ingredients

- 3 ears of fresh corn on the cob, shucked
- 2 tsp jalapeños, finely diced (seeds and membranes removed)
- 1/4 cup red onion, minced
- 1/4 cup fresh cilantro, finely chopped
- Juice from one lime
- 1/2 tsp sea salt

Directions

1. Preheat grill to medium heat.
2. Cook the shucked corn on the preheated grill, turning occasionally, until the corn is tender and specks of black appear on the kernels – about 10 minutes. Set aside until cool.
3. Cut the corn kernels off the corn (here are three easy tips for cutting the kernels off the corn cobs) and put the corn into a bowl.
4. Add the remaining ingredients to the corn and stir until well combined.

Baked Zucchini Fries

Ingredients

- 2 to 3 medium zucchini cut into fries
- 1/4 cup flour
- 1/4 tsp salt
- 1/4 tsp garlic powder
- 1/4 cup Vegan Parmesan cheese (optional)
- 1/2 cup milk (whatever kind you like)
- 1 cup Panko breadcrumbs

Directions

1. Preheat oven to 425F.
2. Line a baking sheet with parchment paper.

3. In shallow bowl or pie plate mix together the flour, salt, garlic powder and optional Vegan Parmesan Cheese.

4. In another bowl pour your milk.

5. In another shallow bowl or pie plate add the bread crumbs.

6. Dip the zucchini into the flour mixture, then into the milk, then into the breadcrumbs and place the zucchini onto the lined baking sheet leaving space between each piece.

7. Bake 20 minutes or until desired crispiness. NOTE: For extra crispiness,

you can finish in the broiler for approximately 2 minutes.

8. Serve with your favorite marinara, dairy-free ranch or tzatziki sauce.

Easy & Healthy Avocado Chicken Salad

Ingredients

- 1 large chicken breast
- salt and pepper
- olive oil
- 1 ripe avocado
- 1 apple
- 1/2 cup celery

- 1/4 cup red onion
- 2 tbsp finely chopped cilantro
- 2 tsp lime juice

Directions

1. Butterfly your chicken by laying the cutlet flat and slicing it parallel with a knife. Season with salt and pepper. Place the chicken breastsinto a lightly oiled skillet over medium-high heat. Cook until brown and opaque throughout, 2-4 minutes each side. Remove from heat and set aside for a few minutes. Finely dice the chicken breast and toss into a large bowl.

2. Dice your veggies. Wash, dry, peel and finely dice your red onion, apple, celery and avocado. Toss into bowl with chicken. Gently mash the avocado until all of the ingredients are mixed well.
3. Sprinkle in cilantro. Add in lime juice and salt and pepper to taste.
4. Serve as a sandwich or on a bed of greens with a little drizzle of olive oil!

Ginger Lemonade

Ingredients

- 1/3 cup honey

- 2 tablespoons fresh ginger root, peeled and grated
- 4 large strips of lemon peel
- 2 medium sprigs fresh rosemary
- Juice of 4 lemons
- Lemon slices (for garnish, optional)
- 1 large sprig fresh rosemary (for garnish, optional)
- Ice, for serving

Directions

1. Combine the honey, ginger, lemon peel and 2 sprigs rosemary in a small pot with 2 cups of water.
2. Bring mixture to a boil, reduce heat and simmer, stirring constantly, for 10 minutes.
3. Remove from heat and let cool, approximately 15 minutes.
4. Once cool, strain mixture into large pitcher. Discard the ginger and rosemary that was left behind in the strainer.

5. To pitcher, add 6 cups cold water and lemon juice. Stir to combine.

6. Serve over ice with small piece of fresh rosemary and lemon slice as garnish (optional)

Delicious Chili-Lime Grilled Corn

Ingredients

- 4 ears of corn, shucked
- 2 tablespoons mayonnaise (try the Liver Doctor's recipe)
- 1 to 2 tablespoons freshly squeezed lime juice

- 1/4 teaspoon chili powder
- Salt & pepper, to taste

Directions

1. Heat grill to medium-high.
2. Place shucked corn onto the grill and cook about 5 minutes until the kernels begin to brown and char.
3. Turn the corn cobs to continue to char. Continue turning every few minutes until all sides are slightly charred.
4. In a small bowl, mix together mayonnaise, lime juice, and chili powder. Taste and add salt and

pepper if needed, adjust flavor to your liking by adding more lime juice or chili powder.

5. Remove corn from grill, spread a light coating of the mayonnaise mixture onto each cob and serve.

Tuscan Vegetable Soup

Ingredients

- 1 (15-ounce) can low-sodium canellini beans, drained and rinsed
- 1 tablespoon olive oil
- 1 cup diced onion (about 1/2 large onion)
- 1/2 cup diced carrots (about 2 carrots)

- 1/2 cup diced celery (about 2 stalks celery)
- 1 1/2 cups zucchini diced (about 1 small zucchini)
- 1 clove garlic, minced
- 1 teaspoon dried thyme leaves
- 1/2 teaspoon dried sage leaves
- 1/2 teaspoon salt
- 1/4 teaspoon freshly ground black pepper
- 32 ounces vegetable broth
- 1 (14.5-ounce) can no salt added diced tomatoes
- 2 cups chopped baby spinach leaves
- 1/3 cup freshly grated Parmesan (optional)

Direction

1. In a small bowl mash half of the beans with a masher or the back of a spoon, and set aside.
2. Heat the oil in a large soup pot over medium-high heat. Add the onion, carrots, celery, zucchini, garlic, thyme, sage, 1/2 teaspoon of salt and 1/4 teaspoon of pepper, and cook stirring occasionally until the vegetables are tender, about 5 minutes.
3. Add the broth and tomatoes with the juice and bring to a boil. Add the mashed and whole beans and the

spinach leaves and cook until the spinach is wilted, about 3 minutes more.

4. Serve topped with Parmesan, if desired.

Homemade Water Kefir Soda

Ingredients

- Water kefir grains
- Room temperature filtered water
- Organic brown sugar
- Organic grape juice

Directions

1. Bring one cup of filtered water to a boil
2. Add 1/2 cup of organic brown sugar stirring until dissolved, then allow to cool completely.
3. In a half gallon jar (64 oz) add 1/2 cup water kefir grains and fill jar half-full with filtered water.
4. Once the brown sugar water is completely cooled add it to the large jar with the water kefir grains and water.
5. Continue to fill the jar with filtered water leaving about a 1 inch

headspace (1 inch of space between the rim of the jar and the top of the liquid).

6. Place the jar lid loosely on top and allow it to ferment on your counter for 24-48 hours (depending on temperature as it will ferment faster in warmer temperatures).

7. After 24 hours sample a taste, if it tastes sweet it needs to ferment longer. Wait another 24 hours.

8. After fermentation is complete, pour 1/4 cup of organic grape juice into four 16 ounce lidded bottles or jars.

9. Fill the bottles the rest of the way by straining the fermented mixture through a very fine mesh strainer or tea towel.
10. Close the lid on the bottles or jars and let sit for another 24 hours (optional). When you open the lid of the bottle or jar, if there isn't a pop or fizzing sound then it probably hasn't fermented enough. If that is the case simply close the lid and let it sit for another day to make it extra bubbly.
11. Pour into a glass and drink.

The Ultimate Healthy Gingersnaps

Ingredients

- 1 3/4 cups (210g) white whole wheat flour or gluten-free flour (NOTE: White whole wheat flour is milled from hard white winter wheat – a lighter-colored grain than traditional red wheat – which yields milder-tasting baked goods. It is not bleached.)
- 1 1/2 tsp cornstarch
- 1 tsp baking powder
- 1 3/4 tsp ground ginger
- 1/4 tsp ground cinnamon
- 1/8 tsp ground nutmeg
- 1/8 tsp ground cloves
- 1/4 tsp salt

- 2 tbsp unsalted butter or coconut oil, melted

- 1 large egg white, room temperature

- 2 1/4 tsp vanilla stevia

- 2 tsp alcohol-free vanilla extract

- 1/4 cup nonfat milk, room temperature

- 1/4 cup unsulphured molasses

- 3 tbsp granulated-style stevia (or more, as needed)

Direction

1. Preheat the oven to 325°F, and line a baking sheet with a silicone baking mat or parchment paper.

2. In a medium bowl, whisk together the flour, cornstarch, baking powder, ginger, cinnamon, nutmeg, cloves, and salt. In a separate bowl, whisk together the butter, egg, vanilla stevia, and vanilla extract. Stir in the milk and molasses. Add in the flour mixture, stirring just until incorporated.

3. Divide the dough into 18 equal portions, and roll each into a ball. Working with one sphere at a time, roll in the granulated-style Swerve until coated. Place onto the prepared baking sheet. Flatten to the desired

width using the flat bottom of a drinking glass. (These cookies don't spread while baking!)

4. Sprinkle the flattened cookie dough with a little more granulated-style Swerve, and gently press it down into the cookie dough with your fingertips. Bake at 325°F for 8-10 minutes. Cool on the baking sheet for 10 minutes before transferring to a wire rack.

www.ingramcontent.com/pod-product-compliance
Lightning Source LLC
Chambersburg PA
CBHW050253220526
45465CB00002B/664